DR. SEBI CURE FOR HERPES

A Comprehensive & Effective Cure Guide for Herpes Virus using best natural therapeutic approaches, tips and remedies

Samuel Lee

©COPYRIGHT 2021-ALL RIGHTS RESERVED.

All rights reserved. The total or partial reproduction of this work, or its incorporation into a computer system, or its transmission in any form or by any means (electronic, mechanical, photocopy, recording or others) is not allowed without the prior written authorization of the owners of copyright. Violation of such rights may constitute a crime against intellectual property.

Legal Notice:

All book content is one's intellectual property and copyrighted. It is only for individual use belongs to the person who wrote/buy it. You have no rights to make changes in it, to sell it, to distribute or rephrase any part of it.

Disclaimer Notice:

The content published in this book is provided "as is" without warranty of any kind, either expressed or implied, including, without limitation, warranties of merchantability, fitness for a particular purpose and non-infringement.

This book may contain advices, opinions and statements from various information providers. It does not represent or endorse the accuracy or reliability of the suggestions, opinions, declarations or other information provided by any information provider, any reader or any other person or entity. Trust in any advice, opinion, statement or other information will also be at the risk and expense of the reader. Neither the owner nor the author will be responsible to the reader or any other person for any inaccuracy, error, omission, interruption, elimination, defect, alteration or use of any content in this document, or for its timeliness or integrity.

Table of Contents

Introduction 5

Dr. Sebi Recommended Medication 21

Dr. Sebi Recommended Natural Products 26

Dr. Sebi Therapeutic Approach 29

Ideal Food To Cure Herpes 38

Herpes Diet Recipes 43

Comprehensive & Useful Tips 83

Conclusion 86

Introduction

Herpes is a widespread infectious disease caused by viruses. Once infected with it, the virus remains unnoticed in the body for a lifetime. If the immune system is weakened, however, it can break out again and cause the typical herpes sores.

Herpes can be caused by viruses. There are different herpes viruses that can cause very different diseases in humans. They are referred to as human herpes viruses, or HHV for short, and are differentiated within this group by numbering from one to eight.

They usually announce themselves hours in advance by tingling, feeling of tension or a slight burning sensation: Cold sores usually appear on the lip of the infected person. But they can also appear on the nose, fingernails, eyes or buttocks. The itchy and painful blisters are caused by type 1 herpes simplex viruses. Normally, the symptoms of the disease are unpleasant, but not dangerous. But especially with certain risk groups such as patients undergoing chemotherapy, newborns or HIV patients, life-threatening complications can arise when a herpes infection breaks out. But even in healthy people, herpes can spontaneously trigger encephalitis, often with irreversible damage.

Once infected with herpes viruses, you will not get rid of them for the rest of your life. Most of the time they are in the idle state. Only when the immune system is weakened, for example in the case of infectious diseases, fever, stress or strong sunlight, the herpes viruses become active again. Most people become infected with herpes before the age of six. In the first few hours after infection, it is decided in each individual infected cell whether the virus will actively multiply or go into dormant state. . The doctor and his team want to understand how this decision is made. These findings could provide new starting points for therapies to combat the herpes viruses.

How herpes viruses take control

What happens when the viruses enter the human body? What tricks do they use to evade the immune system? And how do viruses manage to take command in individual cells? The researchers are looking for answers to these questions. What is certain is that the genetic material of the virus consists of DNA, just like in humans. As soon as the herpes pathogen has penetrated a human cell, it smuggles its genetic material into the cell nucleus.. In the resting state, the virus hides there so that it cannot be recognized and attacked by the infected person's immune system.

The molecular machinery with which genetic information is read from the DNA and transcribed into so-called RNA molecules is located in the cell nucleus. This RNA then determines which proteins the cell makes, for example to promote cell growth. Herpes viruses are able to take control of this machinery. They use the cells to have their own proteins produced in large quantities and to multiply on a massive scale. The cell is ultimately destroyed, releasing thousands of new virus particles in the process.

"Herpes" usually means the typical symptoms caused by the herpes simplex virus (HSV). The viruses of the genus Herpes simplex are again subdivided into type 1 and type 2, i.e. HSV1 and HSV2. The corresponding abbreviation for the human herpes types is HHV1 or HHV2. HSV1 is mainly responsible for cold sores, HSV2, on the other hand, is usually the cause of genital herpes. Ultimately, however, both types of virus can cause herpes in both parts of the body.

Other herpes viruses cause diseases such as chickenpox and shingles (HHV3), glandular fever (HHV4) or three-day fever (HHV6 / 7).

Once infected with the herpes virus, the virus remains in the body for life and can become active again at any opportunity (reactivation).

First herpes infection

As a viral disease, herpes is contagious. It is transmitted from person to person, mainly through smear infection. The herpes virus has to get from the infection site or from the saliva of a sick person to the mucous membranes of a healthy person - for example when kissing or having sexual intercourse. In general, the risk of herpes transmission increases even with close physical contact, so that infection can also take place among children while playing, for example.

Sometimes herpes is passed on indirectly between people or from one part of the body to another. If the sick person scratches the infected area, for example, the herpes viruses get to his hand and can infect other parts of the body or people.

Contagion can also sometimes occur through objects such as used glasses. Herpes, however, needs moisture. If the herpes viruses dry out, they die. According to recent research, the herpes viruses can survive outside the body for up to 48 hours. Since the saliva of an active herpes disease on the lips and mouth is also infected with viruses and is contagious, the herpes viruses can even be transmitted by means of droplet infection in physical proximity. When you speak, tiny droplets of saliva are created that travel short distances in the air and can thus get onto the mucous membranes of other people.

Herpes reactivation

The herpes simplex virus is not completely destroyed by the immune system, but only put into a kind of dormant state (latency). Within certain cells, it remains inactive most of the time and does no harm. Under certain circumstances, the herpes disease can reactivate.

After the first infection with the herpes simplex virus (primary infection), the viruses initially multiply in so-called epithelial cells on the surface of the skin. There they are fought by the immune system, but some of the viruses migrate along nerve fibers to their cell bodies. Here they survive for a lifetime, unnoticed by the immune system. Herpes viruses mainly collect in so-called nerve ganglia, collections of nerve cell bodies.

If the immune system is temporarily or permanently weakened, individual herpes viruses can migrate from the ganglia back to the epithelial cells. There they multiply again and cause the typical symptoms again. How often such reactivations occur varies greatly from person to person. Some people develop herpes several times a year, others are rarely or not at all affected after the primary infection. The genital herpes caused by HSV2 is reactivated more often than the cold sore caused by HSV1.

When is herpes contagious?

Herpes is contagious only during primary infection or reactivation. That is when viruses are excreted. However, the classic symptoms do not always have to be present. In so-called latent infections, those affected excrete viruses, but show no symptoms. If the appropriate precautionary measures are not taken, the risk of herpes transmission increases. Herpes infection is not possible while the virus is in a dormant state.

Incubation period

There are about three to seven days (incubation period) between the infection and the appearance of symptoms; several weeks are also possible.

Who does herpes affect?

Herpes is an extremely contagious disease. According to a study, up to 85 percent of Germans are infected with the type 1 herpes simplex virus. With HSV2, the rate is significantly lower at around 15 percent.

HSV2 mostly causes genital herpes and is mainly transmitted through sexual intercourse. Herpes simplex virus 1, on the other hand, is widespread and is usually passed on within the family as early as infancy or toddler age.

Herpes: symptoms

The typical, painful herpes blisters usually appear on the face (especially on the lip) or in the genital area. In addition, herpes can affect other parts of the body and in rare cases lead to serious complications. In addition, the primary infection with herpes sometimes differs from reactivation.

At first, unspecific complaints (prodromal symptoms) often occur, later the typical symptoms on the skin appear . The first symptoms follow the incubation period and can appear up to two days before the actual illness. General malaise, fatigue, headache , fever and sometimes nausea are typical . During this prodromal phase, there is often an itchy or tingling sensation in the areas where the vesicles eventually develop, even slight pain is possible. The actual herpes outbreak is then accompanied by fluid-filled blisters on reddened skin, swelling and skin damage. One can only speak of "herpes stages" to a limited extent, because the transitions are fluid. Even after vesicles have burst and become encrusted, fresh vesicles can form again.

Herpes in children

Herpes for the first time in children is often more difficult than in adults. The children often feel very miserable, with a high fever, similar to a strong cold or flu . The classic herpes symptoms do not necessarily have to occur, so that herpes in toddlers and children is sometimes not recognized as such, but is taken to be a normal viral infection.

A special form of herpes in children is Gingivostomatis herpetica, in which there is a pronounced infestation in the mouth; adults are also occasionally affected. You can read more about this under " Herpes in the mouth ".

Herpes symptoms when reactivated

In contrast to the primary infection, the initial herpes stage is usually much weaker with a reactivated outbreak and only lasts a few hours. Often those affected have no symptoms at all before the actual herpes symptoms appear. Although the outbreak is often weaker than with the initial infection with herpes, the course and type of symptoms are then the same.

How long does herpes last?

The fluid-filled blisters usually heal again after six to ten days, but the "herpes duration" can also be two or three weeks until they have completely healed. How long the disease lasts also depends on the stage of the disease. In the case of an initial infection, the symptoms are often a bit more persistent; in the case of reactivation, the body's defenses are already familiar with the herpes virus and get the infection under control more quickly.

If the herpes symptoms persist for an unusually long time, there may be a so-called superinfection in addition to an immune deficiency - an additional bacterial infection of the affected areas of the skin. Because the damaged skin is an ideal entry point for bacteria when the body's defenses are weakened.

How long is herpes contagious?

Herpes is contagious when viruses are excreted and fresh blisters can be seen. The greatest risk of herpes infection comes from the liquid in the vesicles, which contains a large number of viruses. As soon as all the blisters are encrusted and no new ones appear, the risk of infection is significantly lower. Nevertheless, small amounts of virus can still be excreted sometime after the herpes crust has fallen off.

Special forms of herpes and complications

Herpes simplex infections typically appear on the lips and genital area. Other parts of the body may also be infected. If the eyes or the brain are affected, there is a risk of serious complications.

Herpes on the skin

The herpes simplex virus can be transmitted from the actual infection site - for example by scratching - to other skin areas. This preferably happens on injured or very thin skin regions. For example, herpes on the eyelid and herpes on the back can occur as well as herpes on the arm or herpes on the finger.

A special case is eczema herpeticatum. This is a large-scale herpes infection with rapidly bursting blisters in those affected who also suffer from skin diseases such as neurodermatitis or psoriasis. A pronounced feeling of illness is typical.

Herpes on the eye

Herpes on the eye is a dangerous special case . A distinction is made between an infection of the cornea (herpes simplex keratitis) and the retina (herpes simplex retinits). While corneal involvement can be caused by external transmission as well as by reactivations, in the case of herpes on the eye with mere retinal involvement, only reactivations are the trigger. Herpes simplex keratitis can usually be treated well by the doctor, but if the retina is affected, there is a risk of blindness in the affected eye. Ocular herpes is a serious complication that needs to be treated as soon as possible.

Herpes encephalitis

Herpes encephalitis (inflammation of the brain) can also trigger the virus, usually HSV1. If herpes is located in the brain, life-threatening complications are possible. At the beginning there is often severe nausea with vomiting and headache, later epileptic seizures, states of confusion and odor disorders can occur before the patient finally falls into a coma. If left untreated, herpes simplex encephalitis is fatal in around 70 percent of cases.

Generalized herpes simplex

Another complication is the generalized form of the disease. The viruses then get into the bloodstream and multiply there excessively (viraemia). Doctors also refer to severe forms as herpes simplex sepsis, i.e. blood poisoning with herpes viruses.

Generalized forms usually only occur in high-risk patients with a severely weakened immune system - for example after chemotherapy or organ transplants.

Genital herpes

Herpes is particularly annoying in the genital area and is usually associated with high levels of shame.

Herpes in the mouth

First-time herpes in children sometimes leads to a widespread infection in the mouth.

Herpes in Pregnancy

There are a few things to consider when it comes to herpes during pregnancy.

Herpes: cause and risk factors

The herpes simplex virus type 1 or type 2 is a relatively large DNA virus that is usually strictly specialized in its host, i.e. humans. Herpes infection does not normally take place from animals to humans or vice versa. The virus is usually transmitted within the family environment as early as childhood.

Children are often in close physical contact, so herpes is particularly contagious with them. Above all, the liquid content of the vesicles ensures infection with herpes, so you should not puncture them.

Risk factors for herpes reactivation

A reactivation of the herpes disease usually occurs when the immune system is weakened or the nerve along which the viruses migrate is irritated. The reasons for this can be varied. Common causes of herpes are:

- Colds and flu-like infections
- Mental and physical stress

- Certain medications, such as cortisone or chemotherapy drugs
- Too much UV light
- Hormonal changes
- Injuries
- Immunodeficiency Disease HIV

Colds weaken the immune system and allow dormant herpes viruses to return to the surface of the skin from the nerve ganglia. The herpes symptoms then often occur together with a fever, which is why one also speaks of "cold sores". However, fever alone does not cause blisters.

Why do you often get herpes after sunburn? Excessive UV radiation irritates not only the skin but also nerves and herpes viruses can be activated. In the same way, skin injuries can promote reactivation.

People with chronically compromised immune systems are also more prone to reactivations with herpes. Triggers of a permanent immune deficiency are, for example, an infection with the immunodeficiency disease HIV or the consequences of chemotherapy. But not everyone who complains "constantly having herpes" must have an immunodeficiency. Some people suffer from reactivation more often than others without a specific reason being found. Stress in particular, be it physical or emotional, seems to favor herpes and frequent reactivations.

Many factors can contribute to the fact that the viral infection keeps flaring up:

- heavy stress on the skin and skin injuries - also from the sun's UV radiation
- a weak immune system with colds and flu or due to previous illnesses
- hormonal changes or fluctuations, such as those caused by the female cycle
- emotional and physical stress

The fluid contained in the vesicles is highly contagious. If they burst, a purulent scab forms, which can sometimes become cracked as it progresses. Only gradually do the blisters heal completely. A herpes attack usually lasts one to two weeks.

Examination and diagnosis

On the basis of the medical history and the symptoms, the doctor can usually easily recognize herpes; a simple visual diagnosis is often sufficient. In rare cases it is helpful to precisely identify the pathogen in the laboratory.

Protection against herpes

Most people have herpes viruses in their bodies. It is therefore particularly important to avoid outbreaks, prevent transmission to other parts of the body and alleviate symptoms.

Because herpes is so easily transmitted, there is no safe protection. Contact with cold sores and herpes ulcers should be avoided - even with your own so as not to transmit viruses, for example, from the lips to the eyes. If you have touched cold sores or sores, thorough hand washing helps.

Condoms only reduce the risk of herpes transmission during sex to a limited extent - for example because they do not cover all regions with cold sores, because the fingers of used condoms transmit herpes viruses to other places or because viruses also occur when kissing, caressing, licking or transferred to other sex practices.

In the case of genital herpes in the last weeks of pregnancy, a caesarean section is recommended to protect the newborn

There is no vaccination against a herpes simplex infection.

Prevent herpes outbreaks

To avoid herpes recurrence, one should

- eat a balanced diet
- get enough sleep
- move regularly
- Avoid stress as much as possible
- Care for the lips (herpes occurs more easily with chapped lips; in strong sunlight, a lip balm with a sufficient sun protection factor is recommended).

If herpes does occur, anti-virus agents should be used at the first sign.

Methods of examination for herpes

The following methods are available to rule out similar diseases or to check herpes viruses for possible drug resistance:

Antibody determination (serology)

If the body is confronted with a pathogen, the healthy immune system forms so-called antibodies, which play an important role in destroying the pathogen. The detection of certain antibodies now indicates a herpes infection, but the result of such tests is not always clear. Especially in the case of immune compromised there are sometimes no herpes antibodies, although the patient is infected.

Antibody determination is helpful in determining the spread of the infection in a population group.

Antigen determination

A much more accurate method with which one can recognize herpes is the detection of so-called antigens. This describes the smallest biological components that stimulate the body's immune system to produce antibodies. Such antigens are usually foreign substances, such as components of viruses or bacteria. The herpes virus also has components that the test can detect.

Direct virus detection with PCR

The most accurate method to reliably detect herpes viruses is to artificially multiply the virus DNA in the laboratory. Even with the smallest amounts of virus, the genetic material of the virus can be reproduced with this method so often that it can finally be detected. This method is called the polymerase chain reaction (PCR).

Growing the herpes viruses

The most complex detection variant is the cultivation of the herpes viruses. To do this, a sample is placed in a nutrient fluid - by adding medication, the reaction of the virus can be tested and therapies adjusted. A distinction between HSV1 and 2 is also possible.

Dr. Sebi Recommended Medication

Dr. Sebi clearly stated that treatment of herpes is mainly supported by antivirals. The pathogens are not destroyed, but you can stop their reproduction. Antivirals help against different types of herpes and usually have the same mechanism of action. The remedies often end in "-ciclovir".

In addition to the antiviral drugs, anti-inflammatory, antiseptic and analgesic preparations can also be used. The herpes is not combated directly, but the remedies work against the symptoms or reduce the external spread of the virus. Some herbs have a pleasantly cooling effect, others help the crusts to detach more quickly.

Possible resistances

Many of the antiviral drugs are used not only to treat herpes simplex, but also for other herpes diseases such as Pfeiffer's glandular fever or herpes zoster. Some are also prescribed for completely different viral diseases. This can promote the development of resistance. This makes herpes viruses resistant to the active ingredients. This can be dangerous for patients if the treatment of complications, such as meningitis caused by herpes viruses or blood poisoning, does not work due to drug resistance. - It is therefore very important to use herpes medication sparingly and responsibly. In many cases, drug therapy is not even necessary, as some herpes diseases heal on their own.

Homeopathy for herpes

Homeopathic remedies can be helpful for all herpes infections. The selection of the right active ingredient depends on the type of herpes and the individual symptoms. Patients who suffer from severe forms of the disease should only take homeopathic medicines in addition to conventional medical treatment. These remedies help, among other things, with herpes infections (selection):

- Apis: For shingles.
- Arsenicum album: For cold sores and shingles.
- Dulcamara: For cold sores and genital herpes.
- Rhus toxicodendron: When cold sores occur during the course of a febrile cold.

Acupuncture for herpes

An important goal in treatment with acupuncture is to create a healthy balance in the patient's energy flow and to loosen possible blockages. In the case of an infectious disease such as herpes, the therapy can, among other things, help to strengthen the body's own defenses. Certain acupuncture points are pierced with the fine needles along the so-called meridians. Depending on the individual symptoms, an experienced acupuncturist will be able to alleviate a herpes disease in many cases and strengthen the immune system.

Herpes in children

Children who develop herpes for the first time suffer from more severe symptoms than adults. They often get a high fever, like a bad cold or flu, and feel very miserable. However, the characteristic herpes symptoms with oozing blisters do not always show up. It happens that the disease is sometimes undiagnosed in both young and older children. Instead, the doctor assumes a normal viral infection. However, there is a special form of herpes that is easy to recognize: the gingivostomatis herpetic. This shows a strong infestation with cold sores in the mouth and throat, which is very painful. Adults can also be affected by the form of herpes, also known as mouth rot. Herpes in the mouth is usually transmitted through a smear infection. The infection does not necessarily have to come from a person with oral herpes. Herpes on the lip can also lead to herpes in the mouth in others. The viruses are mainly found in the fluid in the cold sore and then spread through the saliva. The preferred entry points for the herpes viruses are the corners of the mouth and lips, as the skin there is particularly thin and often has small cracks. - Drug treatment can often reduce the severity of symptoms in mouth herpes but cannot prevent the outbreak. Doctors give pain relievers to young children in particular to make it easier to eat and drink. The viruses are mainly found in the fluid in the cold sore and then spread through the saliva. The preferred entry points for the herpes viruses are the corners of the mouth and lips, as the skin there is particularly thin and often has small cracks. - Drug treatment can often reduce the severity of symptoms in mouth herpes but cannot prevent the outbreak. Doctors give pain relievers to young children in particular to make it easier to eat and drink. The viruses are mainly found in the fluid in the cold sore and then spread through the saliva. The preferred entry points for the herpes viruses are the corners of the mouth and lips, as the skin there is particularly thin and often has small cracks. - Drug treatment can often reduce the severity of symptoms in mouth herpes but cannot prevent the outbreak. Doctors give pain relievers to young children in particular to make it easier to eat and drink.

Herpes in pregnant women

If a herpes disease occurs shortly before the birth, it is possible that the herpes viruses are transmitted from the mother to the child during delivery. Depending on how severe the herpes disease is and whether there is a primary infection or a relapse, the mother can be treated with a virus-inhibiting drug. It may be appropriate to consider a caesarean section. - If there is a likelihood that the newborn has become infected with herpes viruses, an antiviral is usually administered via the vein. This should rule out serious complications such as encephalitis.

Prevent herpes

Since a large part of the population is infected with herpes simplex virus type 1, it can hardly be avoided. The virus is mostly responsible for cold sores, but it can also affect other parts of the body. Many are infected with the herpes virus type 1 in their childhood. However, the transmission of genital herpes (genital herpes, herpes simplex virus type 2) can be prevented by taking appropriate contraceptive measures with condoms. If one is infected with herpes simplex, a strong immune system can protect against frequent reactivations. A healthy lifestyle with a balanced diet, lots of exercise and little stress helps. In the cold season you should take care of your lips, as chapped and chapped lips make it easier for the pathogen to penetrate and thus lead to cold sores. In summer, a sufficient sun protection factor is recommended as a precaution against excessive UV radiation for the lips. An effective vaccination against herpes does not yet exist.

Herpes - ICD code

In medicine, every illness is assigned its own ICD code. The abbreviation ICD stands for International Statistical Classification of Diseases and Related Health Problems. The classification system is recognized worldwide and one of the most important for medical diagnoses. An "infection by herpes viruses (herpes simplex)" is recorded under the ICD code "B00". Entering this code often helps with research on the Internet.

Dr. Sebi Recommended Natural Products

Herpes, also known as a "cold sore ", cold sore is a mild infectious disease. It is caused by a very contagious virus which is transmitted by direct or indirect contact with an infected person. The cold sore is manifested by skin lesions as bubbles, as small bulbs at the mouth. Before the appearance of these lesions, one may feel tingling, itching or a burning sensation on the affected area, as before the appearance of a pimple.

From these first signs, it is essential to act to prevent herpes from "coming out". If solutions based on creams or patches are available in pharmacies, there are also natural remedies which are sometimes sufficient to stop its spread. However, be sure to follow certain hygiene rules to prevent the virus from spreading: always wash your hands before applying a treatment, do not touch the cold sore, do not squeeze it and do not remove dead skin. .

Dry the cold sore with apple cider vinegar

The goal of anti-herpes remedies is to dry out the pimple before it appears, while disinfecting the affected area. Apple cider vinegar helps to dry the skin and accelerate healing. Apply a few drops several times a day with a cotton swab at the first signs of tingling.

In an emergency, apply toothpaste on your pimple

An emergency solution, certainly not very aesthetic, is to apply a little white toothpaste, if possible herbal, on the cold sore. Leave on for a few minutes, then rinse with clean water. This remedy is also well known to fight acne quickly.

Use an ice cube to stop the herpes outbreak

To stop the herpes outbreak in its tracks, apply an ice cube to the itchy area of the mouth. Be sure to wrap the ice cube in a tissue so you don't burn your skin. Hold for ten minutes and repeat the operation two to three times a day.

Use baking soda for cold sores

Are fabricating a paste by diluting a spoonful of coffee baking soda food in warm water. Then apply this mixture twice a day directly on the cold sore. Leave on for half an hour and rinse.

Repel herpes attacks with salt water

If you have the opportunity to go swimming in the sea, take advantage! Otherwise, dilute a little salt in hot water, dip a cotton swab in it and gently apply the soaked tip to the pimples, several times a day.

Garlic clove, a natural antiseptic

Garlic is well known for its natural antiseptic properties. It helps to dry out, while disinfecting the skin. Cut a garlic clove in half and rub half of it on the area to be treated for a few seconds, two to three times a day.

Slow the progression of herpes with milk

Rich in lysine, a component that slows the progression of cold sores, milk is an excellent anti-herpes product. Rub a cotton ball soaked in milk on the area to be treated several times a day. The yogurt can also be used locally and consumed during the period of infection.

Lemon juice to naturally stop infection

This natural antiseptic, rich in vitamin C, helps fight against the herpes virus. Apply a few drops to the pimple three times a day, and take the opportunity to also consume it in lukewarm water to strengthen your immune system.

Dr. Sebi Therapeutic Approach

For herpes treatment a limited number of drugs is only appropriate as specified by Dr. Sebi. In order to have a positive influence on the course of the disease, they must be used as early as possible. In addition to the antiviral agents, painkillers are sometimes used against herpes.

What helps against herpes?

The so-called antivirals play a central role in herpes therapy. These drugs are used by default against various types of herpes and are also used for other viral diseases. There are also other active ingredients that can be used for herpes, but these only affect the symptoms and not the cause.

Medicines used to treat herpes

There are several antiviral drugs that are approved for treating herpes. However, almost all of them have the same mechanism of action. Most active ingredient names end with "-ciclovir". The active ingredients used include, for example, acyclovir, valaciclovir, ganciclovir, valganciclovir and penciclovir. Brivudine is another preparation that can be used to treat herpes, as is zinc sulfate.

If resistance to these agents occurs, Foscarnet can be given as an alternative. All of these active ingredients are so-called antivirals, which means that they cannot destroy the viruses, but only prevent them from multiplying. Medicines that destroy viruses would be called virucides, but there are currently no such preparations.

Other drugs used in herpes treatment

In addition to the antiviral drugs, there are a few others that do not fight herpes directly, but work against its symptoms or reduce the external spread of the virus. For example, anti-inflammatory and pain-relieving preparations are available, but also antiseptic ones that kill the viruses that penetrate the outside world. Some agents have a cooling effect, others can be used to loosen the crusts more quickly.

What helps quickly against herpes?

"What to do with herpes?" Asks everyone who has ever become acquainted with the annoying blisters and of course you want to get rid of the herpes quickly. Unfortunately, the currently known active ingredients for herpes treatment do not work miracles. At best, they shorten the duration of the illness and alleviate the symptoms, but they do not offer reliable, quick help with herpes.

Early herpes treatment works better

The best way to at least accelerate healing is to start therapy as early as possible. Those affected who suffer from herpes reactivations often have a feeling for the first symptoms of an impending outbreak of the disease. If there are unpleasant sensations, itching or pain in the affected area, you already know that it will not be long before the first fluid-filled blisters appear.

This is the best time to start herpes drug treatment. Some patients even report that they can prevent the outbreak of herpes in this way. The fact that only the early use of antivirals has a significant effect on the course of the disease is explained by the way these drugs work: They can only prevent the virus from multiplying, but cannot destroy "finished" viruses.

Possible problems with herpes treatment with medication

Most of the above-mentioned antiviral drugs are not only used for herpes simplex treatment, but also for other herpes diseases such as Pfeiffer's glandular fever or herpes zoster. Some of them are also used in the treatment of viral diseases outside the herpes group.

This can promote the development of resistance, which means that herpes viruses of all groups are increasingly resistant to the active ingredients. In the worst case, the standard active ingredients no longer work in a patient and only expensive alternatives for herpes treatment are still effective.

This may not be a bad thing for the treatment of simple herpes sores on the lip, but it can be dangerous if the therapy fails for complications such as herpes-related encephalitis or blood poisoning due to drug resistance. It is therefore important to use herpes medication sparingly and responsibly. Medicinal herpes treatment is often not necessary at all, since the herpes would heal after a certain period of time without any further action.

Which treatment for which herpes?

Herpes outbreaks can occur in almost any part of the body, with the face and genital area being the preferred areas for herpes simplex viruses. Herpes simplex viruses of type 1 (HSV1) are usually responsible for infections in the face, for example on the lip or nose, and in the genital area mostly type 2 viruses (HSV2). The antivirals act equally on HSV1 and HSV2, but there are special features in herpes treatment depending on the manifestation.

What to do about herpes on the lip

In most cases, cold sores are harmless even without medication. However, timely antiviral therapy reduces the duration of symptoms such as itching and pain by 20 to 30 percent because it weakens the outbreak of the herpes. Creams that contain acyclovir or penciclovir can help, for example. Studies have not yet sufficiently clarified whether ointments containing zinc sulfate are also effective.

Antivirals are the only thing that helps against herpes on the lip, at least they can shorten the outbreak. The creams for herpes treatment can be applied externally to the affected area. This means that there are fewer side effects. Creams against herpes usually contain additional substances that allow the antiviral active ingredients to penetrate the tissue more quickly. It is recommended to use it up to five times a day for about five to seven days. The creams should not be used in the mouth, on the mucous membrane of the vagina or on the eyes.

Acyclovir and some other antivirals used to treat herpes on the lip can also be given in tablet form. In the case of very pronounced symptoms or complications of the cold sore, intravenous administration of these active ingredients can also be useful.

Finally, there are also herpes patches that are free of active ingredients and that only create a moisture cushion over the cold sore and thus curb the external spread of the virus via smear infection. Since there is no antiviral active component, this does not reduce the duration of the illness.

What helps with herpes in the genital area?

To help against herpes in the genital area, antivirals are mainly used in tablet form. Topical ointments or creams with antiviral active ingredients are only recommended for mild outbreaks of genital herpes.

When genital herpes appears for the first time, tablets are given three to five times a day for at least one week, depending on the concentration of the active ingredient. In severe cases, such as when the patient has a pronounced immune deficiency, the herpes medication must be brought into the bloodstream via the veins . The active ingredients used for intravenous infusion are acyclovir, famciclovir, and valaciclovir.

How to treat herpes in the mouth

Of herpes in the mouth (aphthous stomatitis) Children are mostly affected. Because of the severe pain in the entire mouth and throat, they often refuse to eat with this form of herpes. So what can be done to make the child eat again?

On the one hand, there are gels and creams that contain locally anesthetic agents such as lidocaine and can be applied directly to the diseased mucous membrane in the oropharynx. However, when they come into contact with the tongue, they also suppress the sense of taste. On the other hand, classic pain relievers from the group of non-steroidal anti-inflammatory drugs are available, such as ibuprofen or paracetamol . Both also have an antipyretic effect. Such pain relievers should always be used in children with caution and only on medical advice.

Suitable foods

When choosing food, you should make sure that it does not irritate the oral mucosa as much as possible. Drinks are best given chilled and should not contain acids. Fruit juices are therefore not a good choice, clear water, milk or chamomile tea are better suited. Even solid food causes the least pain if it is pH-neutral, cool and of the softest possible consistency. On the other hand, acidic foods such as tomato sauce or food that is too dry such as rusks or biscuits would irritate the areas affected by the herpes.

Herpes treatment with antivirals is not absolutely necessary for stomatitis aphtosa. Since antiviral drugs are also associated with side effects and children are generally more sensitive to them, their use should always be carefully considered. If the doctor decides, for example because the herpes outbreak is very strong, acyclovir is the drug of choice, either as a tablet or intravenously.

Herpes Treatment During Pregnancy

What can you do about herpes if the patient is pregnant? Can antivirals be used during pregnancy or do they harm the child? These questions are of course of concern to an expectant mother if she has a herpes outbreak during pregnancy.

The known antivirals are not officially approved for use during pregnancy. At least for the active ingredient acyclovir, the observations to date have not shown any negative effects for mother or child.

Whether medicinal herpes treatment is necessary during pregnancy depends on the manifestation of the herpes, at what point in pregnancy the herpes occurs and whether it is a first-time infection or a reactivation. The real danger of herpes during pregnancy is possible transmission to the child. Therefore, especially a genital herpes of the mother is dangerous for the child. Other manifestations such as herpes on the face play almost no role in the transmission to the child.

An initial infection with genital herpes poses a greater risk during pregnancy than reactivations. In addition, the closer the occurrence of the herpes is to the due date, the greater the risk of transmission to the child. Because a large part of the contagion happens during childbirth.

If a reactivated genital herpes occurs in the first or second trimester of pregnancy, medication is usually avoided, while an initial infection in this phase of pregnancy often requires herpes treatment with acyclovir in tablet form or intravenously. If the mother is infected for the first time in the first or second trimester, acyclovir can be given three times a day as a preventive measure from the 36th week of pregnancy. With such a suppression therapy one tries to prevent the occurrence of herpes lesions during the birth and thus to protect the child from infection.

Treatment of initial infections in the last trimester of pregnancy

If herpes symptoms appear in the genital area in the last trimester of pregnancy and it is an initial infection, a caesarean section must be considered. Especially if the herpes breaks out in the last six weeks before the birth, the risk of virus transmission to the child during vaginal birth is otherwise very high. If a caesarean section is actually necessary, but cannot be performed for certain reasons, not only the mother is given acyclovir for herpes treatment, but also the newborn immediately after birth.

What else you should know about herpes treatment

Some people suffer from herpes reactivations very often, sometimes several times a year. In such cases, suppression therapy can often help. For this, the patient receives a low dose of an antiviral continuously for months or even years. Many sufferers can get rid of the typical symptoms of herpes for a long time.

Wrong tips against herpes

By the way, caution is advised with many forum tips against herpes. For example, it is said that if you puncture the vesicles, the herpes will go away quickly ". On the contrary, this ensures an increased release of the virus and thus an increased risk of infection. If the usual herpes treatment is not an option for you, you should rather ask a doctor or pharmacist for advice.

Ideal Food To Cure Herpes

Herpes viruses often "sleep" in the spinal cord for a long time after being infected and multiply suddenly when the immune system is weakened. Then they cause the typical painful blisters.

The right diet can support the immune system. Anyone who is overweight should reduce their abdominal girth, because the belly fat forms inflammatory messengers and thus weakens the immune system. An anti-inflammatory diet is generally recommended - with emphasis on vegetables, with good fats and sufficient protein. An important component in this is largely avoiding sugar in order not to indirectly feed the herpes viruses.

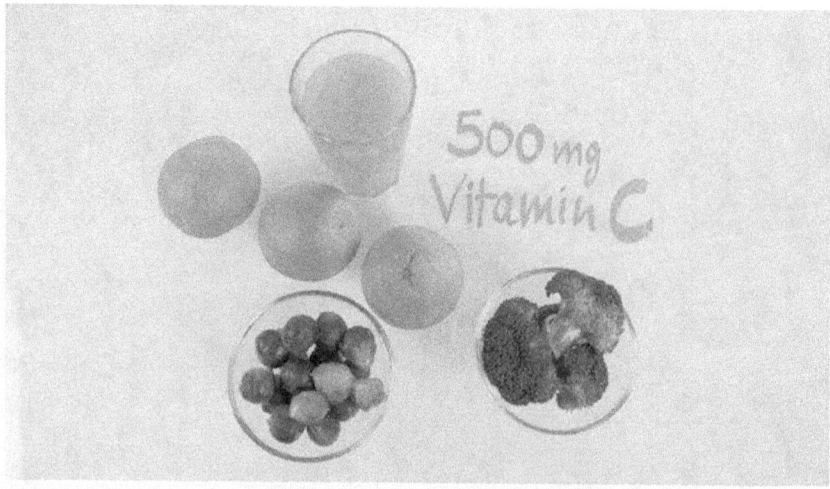

Daily dose of vitamin C: juice from three oranges, 200 g Brussels sprouts, 200 g broccoli.

The aim should always be to supply the necessary vital substances directly with the food and not as a dietary supplement. Because the body can better absorb and process these substances in their natural composite. To strengthen the immune system, vitamin C, zinc and magnesium as well as the amino acids (protein building blocks) lysine and arginine are particularly important.

Ratio of lysine and arginine

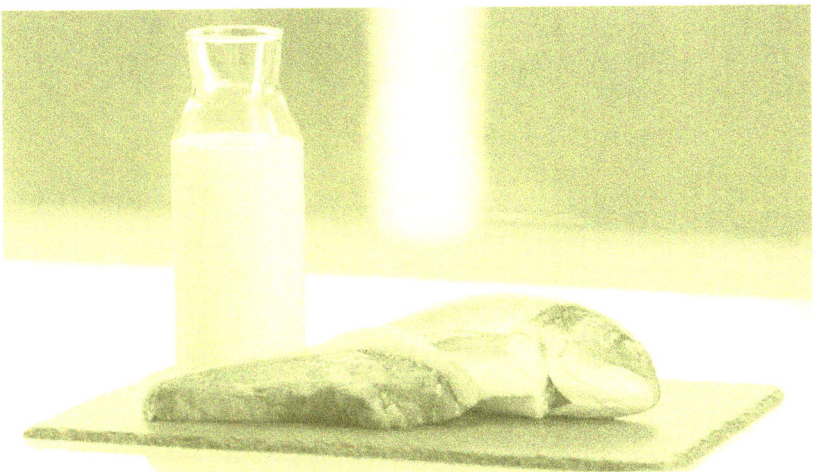

Animal foods are very good sources of lysine.

A healthy person needs the amino acids arginine and - as an opponent - lysine in a balanced ratio. Arginine supports functions of the immune system and also seems to cause improved fat burning and performance. But: arginine also supports the multiplication of herpes viruses - lysine, on the other hand, slows them down. Lysine is an essential amino acid, so we have to get it from food, the body cannot produce it itself. Among other things, he needs lysine for wound healing and cell division. Studies suggest that lysine also makes people less susceptible to stress. However, the disadvantage of long-term very high doses of lysine is that it can apparently increase blood pressure.

Since lysine is mainly found in animal foods, vegans have a harder time meeting their needs. It should also be noted that some good natural mineral sources such as wheat germ, pumpkin seeds and oatmeal are also rich in arginine.

The most important tips:

- **Calm and regular eating,** three-meal structure.
- **If you are overweight: reduce your waist circumference.** Belly fat produces numerous hormones - including inflammatory messengers that put a strain on the immune system. Intermittent fasting can help with weight loss .
- **Refraining from sugar to strengthen the immune system:** if possible, no sweets, pastries, sweet dried fruits; especially avoid chocolate. Bitter substances from the pharmacy help against hunger for sweetness .
- **Carbohydrates in moderation,** preferably use old types of grain: spelled, emmer, einkorn and sham grains such as buckwheat, quinoa.
- Eat high in lysine - up to 30 mg lysine per kilo of body weight per day - and low in arginine.

- **Prefer foods rich in lysine:** eggs, **lean** meat, fish (except tuna); Tofu, cottage cheese, skimmed quark, parmesan, gouda, cow's milk; smaller amounts also in fruit and vegetables - especially in legumes: beans, lentils, chickpeas, soy.
- **Avoid foods rich in arginine:** nuts, chocolate, wheat germ; also tuna, oat flakes, unpeeled rice, whole wheat pasta / bread, peas.
- **Correctly dose protein intake:** a total of 1 gram per kilo of body weight per day - dairy products (e.g. porridge with rice flakes and milk or breakfast quark in the morning); sea fish several times a week (also provides omega-3 fatty acids); Legumes (little peas); also like algae. Nuts are rich in protein, but should be avoided in a sensitive phase!
- **Use good oils:** rapeseed oil, linseed oil, olive oil, walnut oil; vegetable fats such as avocado.
- **Vitamins and minerals to strengthen the immune system:** 500 vitamin C, 15 mg zinc and 300 to 500 mg magnesium daily.
- **Sources of Vitamin C:** Sea buckthorn juice, kale, paprika, broccoli, Brussels sprouts, kiwi, lemons, oranges, grapefruit, sauerkraut.
- **Magnesium sources:** for example spinach, berries, bananas, amaranth, quinoa, soybeans, fish.
- **Sources of zinc:** for example liver, yeast flakes, soybeans, lentils, quinoa.

- **Drink a lot:** at least 2 liters per day of water (still mineral water), unsweetened tea (e.g. sage, chamomile, thyme) or broth; do not drink coffee with meals.

Herpes Diet Recipes

Avocado spelled pizza

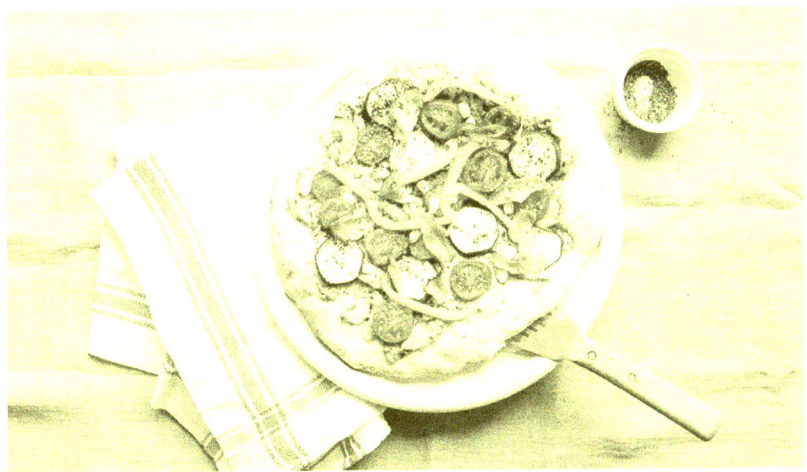

Ingredients for the dough (for a tray):

- 250 g quark
- 400 g spelled flour
- 6-7 tbsp olive oil
- 1 pinch of salt
- 1 packet of baking powder
- 2-3 (depending on size) eggs

Put all the ingredients - quark and eggs at room temperature - in a bowl and knead with your hands. Then set aside for at least a quarter of an hour and let rest.

Preheat the oven to 200 degrees. Line a baking sheet with

parchment paper. Sprinkle some flour on the work surface, roll out the dough and place on the baking sheet.

Ingredients for the sauce:

- 2 avocados
- 2 tbsp olive oil
- 1 tbsp water
- 1 squirt of lemon juice
- if you like: 1-2 cloves of garlic
- oregano

Halve and core the avocados and spoon the pulp into a bowl. Add the remaining ingredients and mix with a hand mixer. Spread the avocado sauce on the pizza dough.

Ingredients for the topping (as desired):

- 300 g tomatoes
- 1 onion
- 100 g mushrooms
- 1 small zucchino
- 100 g cooked ham
- if you like: 1 handful of grated cheese

Wash or clean the vegetables and mushrooms and cut into fine slices. Cut the ham into fine strips. Place everything on the pizza, sprinkle with 1 handful of grated cheese as desired and bake in the oven for 10-15 minutes.

Nutritional values per serving (one tray corresponds to 6 servings): 556 kcal, 24 g protein, 27 g fat, 53 g carbohydrates, 7 g fiber

Bamboo bread (low carb)

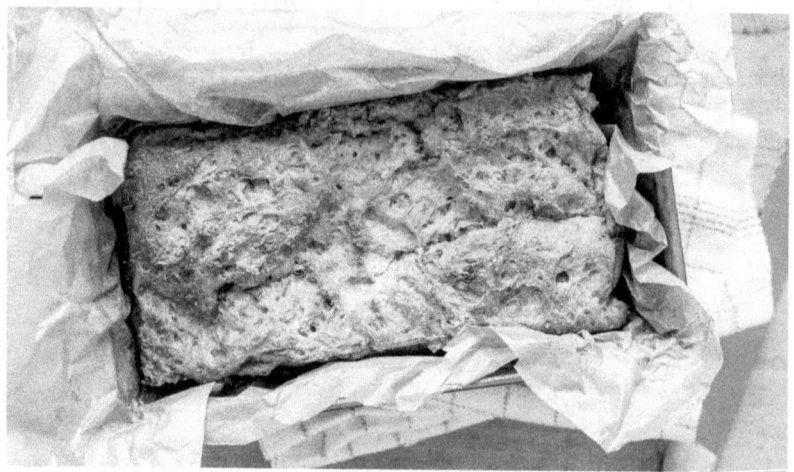

Ingredients for 1 bread (about 12 slices):

- 150 g onions
- 1 tbsp olive oil
- 250 g low-fat quark
- 2 eggs
- 80 g of oat bran
- 25 g bamboo fibers
- 30 g de-oiled gold flaxseed flour
- 1 teaspoon of tartar baking powder
- 1 teaspoon salt

Preheat the oven to 175 degrees (convection).

Peel the onions and cut into cubes. Heat the oil in a pan and fry the onion cubes gently for 5 to 6 minutes.

Then mix the onions well with all the other ingredients in a mixing bowl. Butter a rectangular baking pan or line it with parchment paper. Pour in the batter and bake for 30-35 minutes. Let cool down well before turning over.

Nutritional values per slice (with 12 slices):
63 kcal, 3 g fat, 4 g carbohydrates, 5 g protein, 4 g fiber, 0.4 BE

Bream from the tray with vegetables

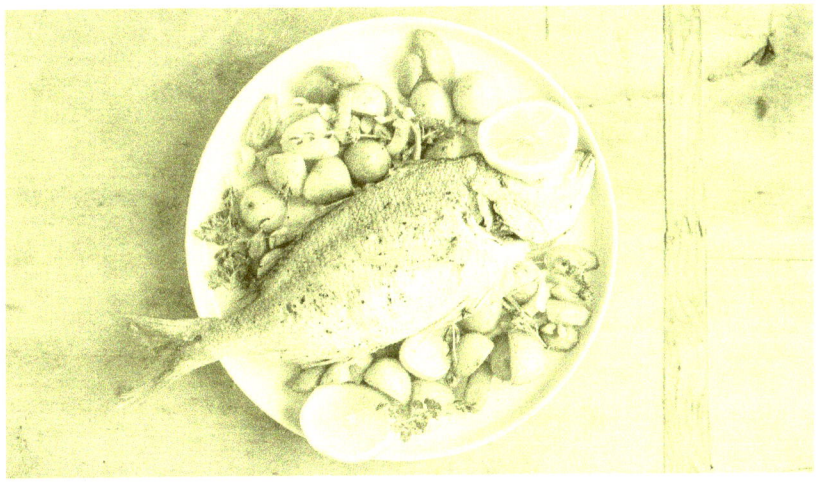

Ingredients:

- 400 g(with green) fennel
- 250 g(in a bunch) carrots
- 250 g small waxy (e.g. triplets) potatoes
- 1 tsp Fennel seeds
- salt

- (from the mill) pepper
- 2 tbsp olive oil
- 1 ready-to-cook bream
- 1 tbsp Lemon juice
- 4 toes garlic
- 2 tsp butter
- for the tray: a little olive oil

Preheat the oven to 220 degrees top / bottom heat (convection 200 degrees). Grease a baking sheet.

Clean and wash the fennel and put the delicate greens aside. Halve the fennel, remove the hard stalk and cut the halves into 1 cm wide wedges. Clean, peel and halve the carrots lengthways. Wash the potatoes, dry them and cut them in half or into quarters depending on the size.

Spread the fennel, carrots and potatoes on the tray. Crush the fennel seeds in a mortar. Season the vegetables with fennel seeds, salt and pepper and drizzle with the olive oil. Cook in the oven on the middle rack for about 15 minutes.

In the meantime, wash the bream inside and out, pat dry, acidify with lemon juice, if desired, and season with salt and pepper. Peel the garlic cloves, cut into slices and pour into the bream. After 10 minutes of cooking, place the fish on top of the vegetables and cover with flakes of butter. Cook the bream and vegetables in the oven on the middle rack for about 25 minutes. Take out of the oven and distribute on plates, serve sprinkled with the chopped fennel leaves.

Nutritional values (per serving):
500 kcal, 39 g protein, 22 g fat, 33 g carbohydrates, 9 g fiber, 3 BE

Emmer rolls

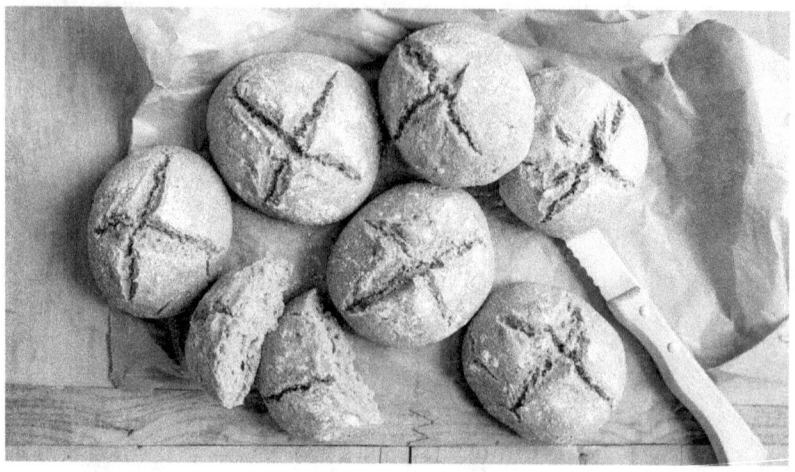

Ingredients (for 8 rolls):

- 300 ml of water
- 20 g yeast
- 10 g of salt
- 500 g emmer flour
- 1 tbsp oil

Mix lukewarm water and yeast together until the yeast has completely dissolved. Then add salt, flour and oil. Knead everything carefully. Let the dough rise in a warm place for at least 1 hour, preferably 2 hours. During the walking phase, the dough should be pulled up and folded up once or twice without much effort.

Preheat the oven to 180 degrees top / bottom heat. Divide the dough into 8 equal parts and form very loose rolls, dust with flour if desired and cut into them. Do not press or knead too hard. Let the rolls rise until the oven has reached the required temperature.

Then bake for about 20 minutes. If possible, switch on a burst of steam at the oven, or alternatively pour a shot glass of water on the bottom of the hot oven to generate steam. This will make the rolls crispier.

Tip:

The rolls can be frozen very easily.

The grain emmer has a favorable ratio of the amino acids lysine and arginine. Dough made from emmer flour must be processed gently, so it should only be kneaded slowly, not very intensively and only until a well-stretchable dough is formed. The dough also takes significantly longer to rise nicely.

Nutritional values per bread roll:
222 kcal, 10 g protein, 3 g fat, 39 g carbohydrates, 6 g fiber, 3.25 BE

Fruity algae smoothie

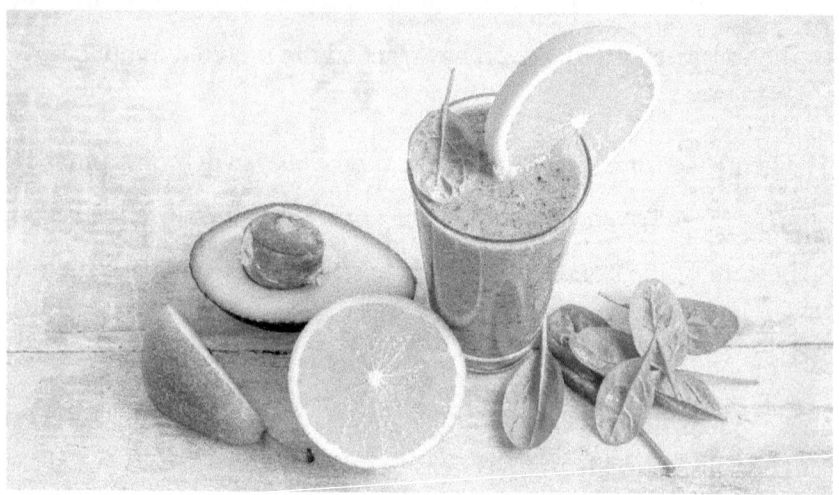

Ingredients:

- 2 handfuls Baby spinach
- 1 handful Lamb's lettuce
- alternatively: kale
- 1 banana
- 0.5 avocado
- 1 pear
- 1 orange
- 1 tsp Coconut oil
- 1 tsp Chlorella powder
- 300 ml Coconut water

Wash and clean the spinach and lamb's lettuce. Peel banana and cut into pieces. Peel the avocado, remove the stone and cut the flesh into small pieces. Wash the pear well, remove the core and cut into pieces with the skin. Squeeze the orange.

Put together with the other ingredients in a blender and mix vigorously.

Nutritional information (per serving):
254 kcal, 13 g fat, 30 g carbohydrates, 4 g protein, 7 g dietary fiber, 2.5 BE

Baked mushrooms & cream cheese

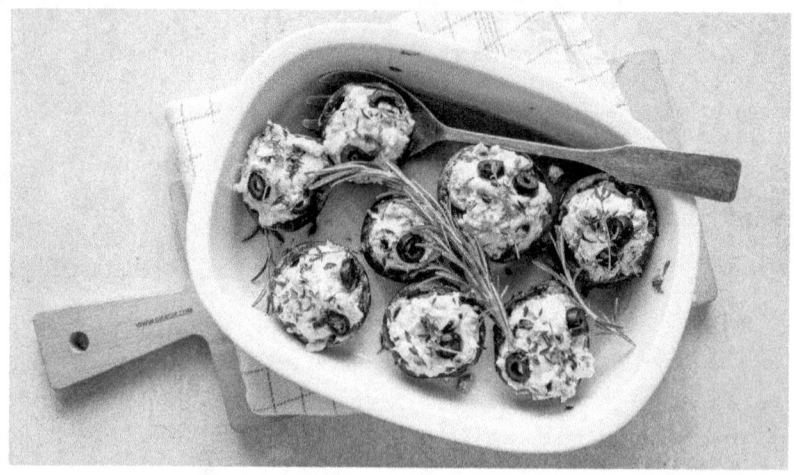

Ingredients:

- 30 g Alaska pollock
- 1 splash Lemon juice
- 10 large mushrooms
- 4 tsps charz (pitted) olives
- 300 g cream cheese
- 2 tbsp olive oil
- salt
- pepper
- at will: Italian herbs
- some chili powder

Preheat the oven to 200 degrees top and bottom heat (180 degrees convection) or heat up the garden grill.

Rinse the fish fillet, pat dry, cut into fine schnitzel and mix with lemon juice. Cleaning mushrooms, detach the stems and chop them into small cubes. Olive cut into thin slices.

Mix the cream cheese with the finely chopped mushroom stalks, olive rings, saithe schnitzel and oil. Season with salt, pepper and chili powder. Pour the cream cheese mixture into the mushrooms and place the mushrooms in a baking dish or grill tray. Cook about 20 minutes.

Nutritional information per serving:
663 kcal, 60 g fat, 5 g carbohydrates, 25 g protein, 3 g dietary fiber, 0.4 BE

Granola (crunchy muesli) with banana

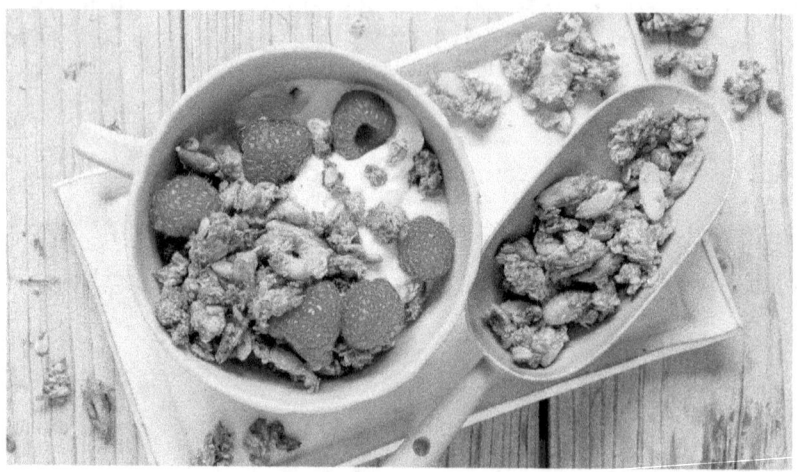

Ingredients for 12 servings (approx. 600 g):

- 2 ripe bananas
- 4 tbsp coconut oil
- 1 teaspoon ground vanilla
- 1 teaspoon cinnamon
- 2 pinches of salt
- 100 g sunflower seeds
- 50 g puffed amaranth
- 200 g flaked almonds
- 50 g desiccated coconut
- 100 g crispy gluten-free oat flakes
- alternatively: spelled flakes

Pre heat the oven to 180 degrees celcius. Line a baking sheet with parchment paper. Peel and roughly dice the bananas. Puree the oil, vanilla and salt in a tall mixing beaker with a hand blender.

Mix the sunflower seeds, amaranth, almonds, desiccated coconut and oat flakes in a bowl. Add the banana puree with a wooden spoon and mix well.

Spread the mixture evenly on the baking sheet and bake in the oven on the lower rack for 25-30 minutes. Mix well every 8 minutes so that the granola browns evenly.

Take the granola out of the oven and let it cool completely on the tray. Then fill into a tightly fitting jar or glass for storage.

To serve, fill approx. 50 g granola per person into bowls. For example, serve with around 200 g (vegan) yogurt and 125 g raspberries or blueberries.

Nutritional values per serving of granola (50 g):
approx. 255 kcal, 18 g fat, 15 g carbohydrates, 8 g protein, 4 g fiber

Mutton pilaf with vegetables and rice

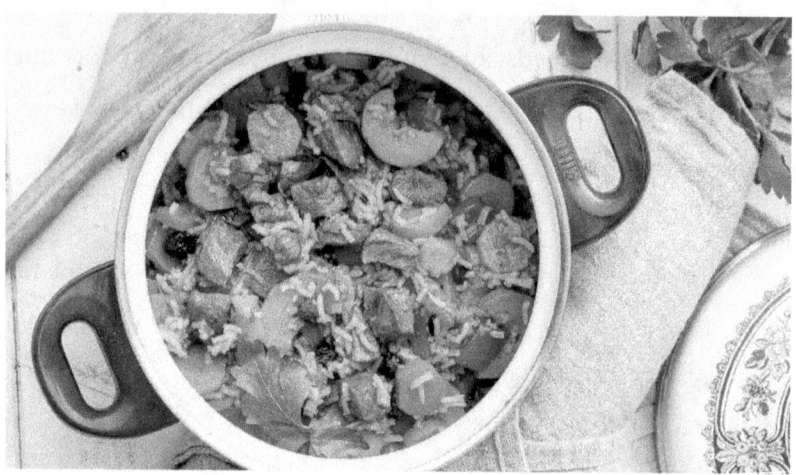

Ingredients:

- 3 Onions
- 6 toes garlic
- 500 g(from shoulder or leg) mutton
- alternatively: lamb
- 1 tspTomato paste
- Paprika powder
- salt
- pepper
- 150 gWhole grain basmati rice
- 6thCarrots
- 2 pods red pepper
- 2Beefsteak tomatoes
- 1 smaller Zucchino

- 2 tbsp olive oil
- alternatively: coconut oil
- 1 l Vegetable broth
- alternatively: lamb stock
- 1 smalle Apple
- 30 g Raisins
- as desired: parsley or coriander

Peel the onions and garlic. Cut the onions into strips, finely chop the garlic. Wash the meat and chop it roughly.

Heat oil in a pot. Fry the meat in it in portions and remove it. Finally, add the onions and garlic to the saucepan and sauté briefly. Add the meat again, dust with paprika powder and season with salt and pepper. Stir in the tomato paste and deglaze everything with the broth. Cover and simmer over low heat.

In the meantime, peel the carrots and cut into slices or cubes. Halve the peppers, remove the core, wash and cut into large cubes. Score the beefsteak tomatoes crosswise and scald them with boiling water so that the skin loosens. Peel off the skin, remove the stalk and dice the tomatoes. Wash and clean the zucchino, halve lengthways and cut into slices.

Wash the rice in a sieve under cold running water and allow to drain. Peel the apple and dice it finely.

After about 20 minutes of braising time, add the rice to the meat, close the lid and bring to the boil, then continue to braise. 10 minutes later add the chopped vegetables, apple and raisins. Let everything simmer gently for about 20-25 minutes. Season to taste with salt and pepper and, if desired, with chopped fresh herbs.

Nutritional values (per serving):
approx. 493 kcal, 34 protein, 15 g fat, 54 g carbohydrates, 11 g fiber, 4.5 BE

Kidney bean patties

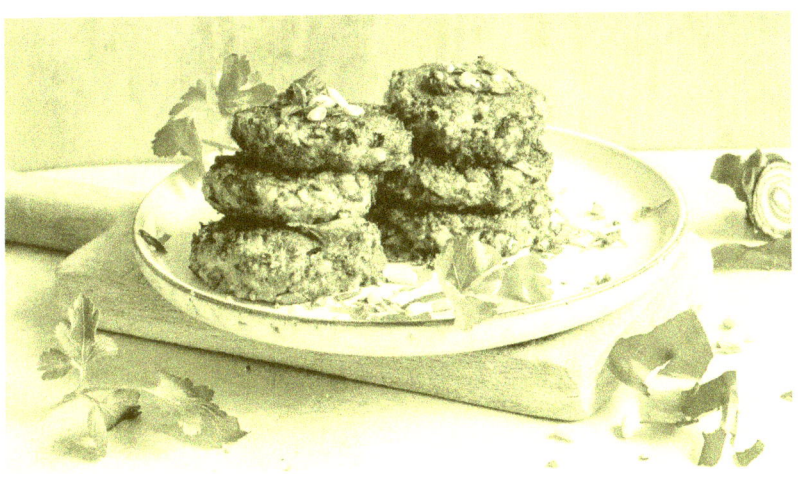

Ingredients:

- 1 Red onion
- 1 toe garlic
- 240 g(Drained weight, from the jar) boiled kidney beans
- 2 tbsp fine oatmeal
- 2 tbspPine nuts
- 2 tbsp parsley
- 1 tsp dried marjoram
- 1 tsp smoked paprika powder
- from the mill: colored pepper
- sea-salt
- 2 tbsp olive oil

Peel and finely chop onions and garlic. Drain the beans in a colander, place in a bowl and mash with a fork. Put briefly in a blender together with the oat flakes. Mix the mass with onions and garlic. Roast pine nuts in a pan for about 3 minutes, chop and fold in. Wash and finely chop the parsley and add to the mass. Season with marjoram, paprika powder, pepper and a little salt.

Use your hands to form around 6 patties from the mixture. Heat the olive oil in a pan and fry the patties on each side for about 4 minutes over medium heat.

Nutritional values (per patty):
approx. 106 kcal, 6 g fat, 9 g carbohydrates, 5 g protein, 4 g fiber, 0.7 BE

Nutritional values (per serving):
approx. 318 kcal, 18 g fat, 27 g carbohydrates, 15 g protein, 12 g fiber, 2.1 BE

Scrambled coconut eggs with seaweed

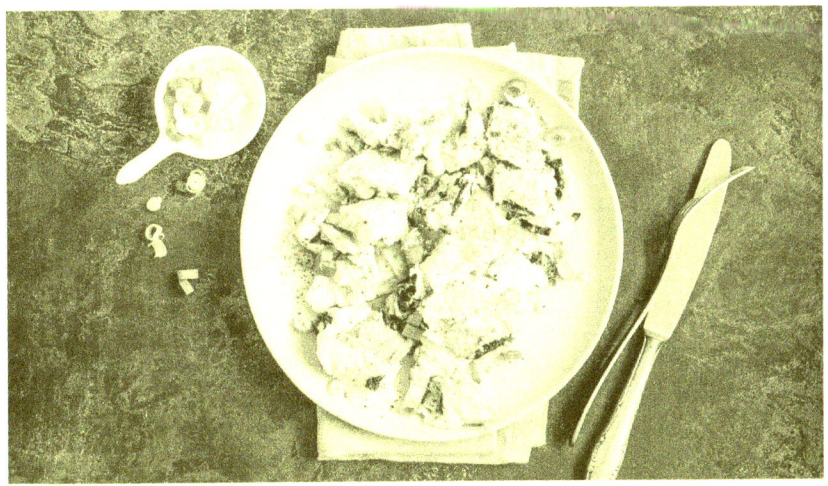

Ingredients:

- 2 spring onions
- 1 sheet Nori
- 4th Eggs
- salt
- pepper
- 1 pinch ground chilli
- 1 tsp Coconut oil

Wash and clean the spring onions and cut into fine rings. Cut the nori seaweed into small squares with the scissors. Whisk the eggs in a bowl, season with salt, pepper and chilli and let the algae soak for about 10 minutes.

Heat the coconut oil in a pan, add the egg mixture to the pan and let it set over a mild heat while stirring.

Chia rolls, for example, go well with it.

Tip:

Fresh and dried algae can be found in Asian supermarkets. People with thyroid problems should consider the sometimes very high iodine content when consuming algae. It is best to only use products for which the iodine content is declared on the packaging, and only in small quantities as a vegetarian alternative to sea fish. You can reduce the iodine content of algae by soaking the algae in water for several hours.

Nutritional values (per serving):
225 kcal, 16 g fat, 5 g carbohydrates, 15 g protein, 1 g fiber, 0.5 BE

Mexico stir-fry vegetables with tofu

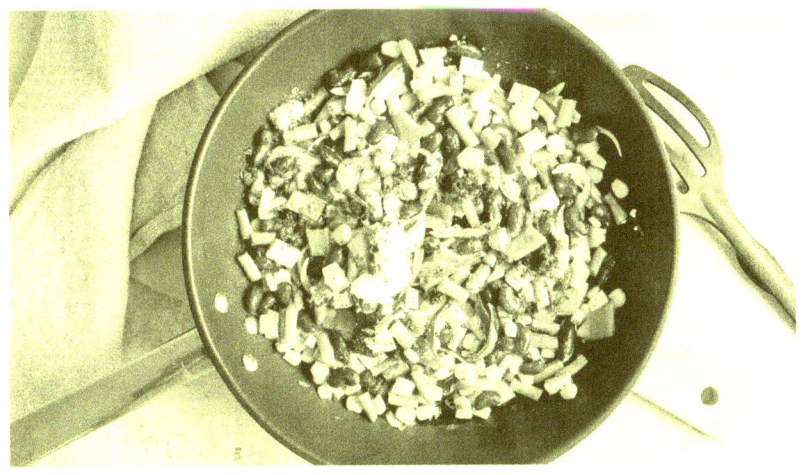

Ingredients:

- 150 g tofu
- 1 packFrozen Mexico vegetables
- 1 tbsp Rape seed oil
- 1 tbspcream cheese
- 1 tbsp Frozen parsley

Cut the tofu into cubes. Fry the ready-to-cook vegetables with the rapeseed oil in a pan and add the tofu. Fry for 4-5 minutes over medium heat. Finally stir in the cream cheese and season with frozen herbs.

Nutritional values (per serving):
307 kcal, 15 g fat, 22 g carbohydrates, 20 g protein, 9 g fiber, 2 BE

Nori roll with avocado

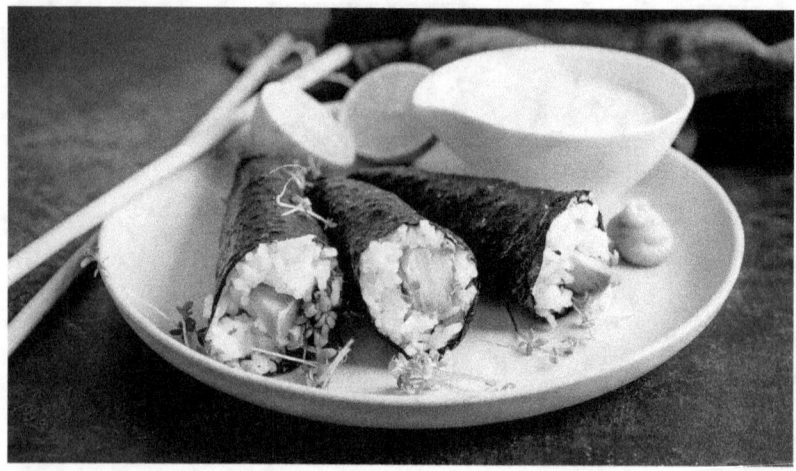

Ingredients for the sushi rice:

- 80 g sushi rice
- alternatively: jasmine or basmati rice
- 160 ml of water
- 1 tbsp rice vinegar
- 1 tbsp mirin
- 0.5 tsp coconut blossom sugar
- salt

The rice is easy to prepare the day before. To do this, rinse the sushi rice in a fine sieve with cold water until the water runs clear, then drain in the sieve for about 20 minutes. Bring to the boil with the water in a saucepan and cook for 2 minutes over a medium heat, then cover and leave to soak on the switched off hotplate for 20 minutes.

Open the lid, cover the rice with a clean tea towel and let stand for another 10 minutes.

Put rice vinegar, mirin, coconut blossom sugar and a little salt in a saucepan and heat, but do not boil. Stir until the sugar and salt have dissolved. Put the sushi rice in a bowl and pick a little apart. Mix in the vinegar mixture and let the rice cool down completely. Cover with a damp cloth until further processing.

Ingredients for the nori (for 8 rolls):

- 160 g cooked sushi rice
- 1 fresh egg
- 120 ml sesame oil
- salt
- 1 organic lime
- 1 tbsp soy sauce
- 1 teaspoon of sugar
- 1 tbsp mirin
- alternatively: lime juice
- 1 avocado
- 1 bowl of cress
- 4 sheets of nori
- 2 tsp wasabi

Wash the lime with hot water and finely grate the peel. Squeeze out and measure 3 tablespoons of juice. Break the egg. Put together with sesame oil, ½ teaspoon salt, lime zest and juice, soy sauce, rice wine and sugar in a tall container. Slowly process with a hand blender into a creamy, thick mayonnaise. Do not stir with the hand blender, just move it slowly up and down. Chill the finished mayonnaise.

Peel the avocado and cut into 8 wedges. Cut the cress from the bed. Halve the nori sheets crosswise. Divide rice into 8 servings.

Place one nori sheet across the work surface. Put a portion of rice in the middle of the leaf, place 1 piece of avocado with a little wasabi on top and cover with cress. Place the left corner of the algae sheet over the filling and roll everything up in the shape of a bag towards the unoccupied corner. Finally, drizzle with the homemade mayonnaise.

Tip:

The vegetarian rolls can be varied with fried shrimp or tuna as desired.

Fresh and dried algae can be found in Asian supermarkets. People with thyroid problems should pay attention to the sometimes very high iodine content when consuming algae! It is best to only use products for which the iodine content is declared on the packaging, and only in small quantities as a vegetarian alternative to sea fish. You can reduce the iodine content of algae by soaking the algae in water for several hours.

Nutritional values (per roll):
221 kcal, 20 g fat, 9 g carbohydrates, 2 g protein, 2 g fiber, 1 BE

Parmesan crackers with herbs

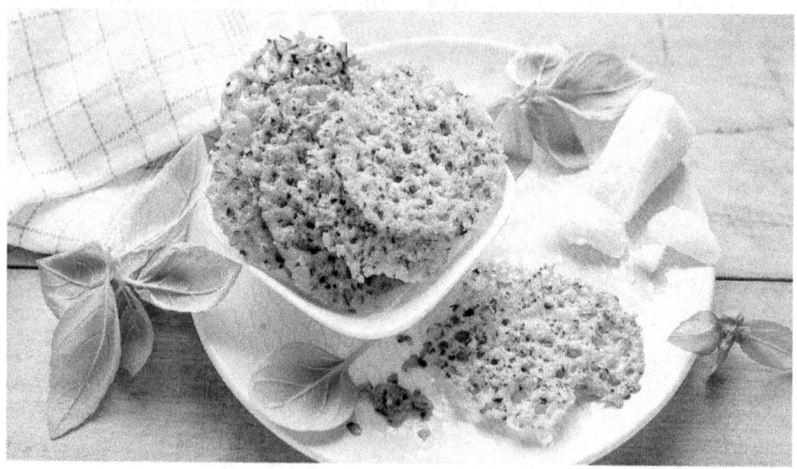

Ingredients (for about 15 pieces):

- 100 g parmesan cheese
- 1 level teaspoon dried Italian herbs or herbs from Provence

Preheat the oven to 200 degrees top / bottom heat.

Grate the parmesan and mix well with the dried herbs of Provence. Line a baking sheet with parchment paper.

Use a tablespoon to place about 15 small heaps of the parmesan mixture on the baking sheet - not too close together. Flatten the piles a little with the back of the spoon.

Then bake on the middle rack for 7–9 minutes until golden. The crackers are good when the edge is starting to brown and the center is still golden yellow. Let the tray cool down for at least 10 minutes, after which the crackers can be easily removed from the paper.

Nutritional values per piece (at 15 pieces):

26 kcal, 2 g fat, 0 g carbohydrate, 2 g protein, 0 g fiber, 0 BE

Tip:

The crispy crackers taste great as an accompaniment to soups and starters as well as as a small snack

Mushroom soup with seaweed

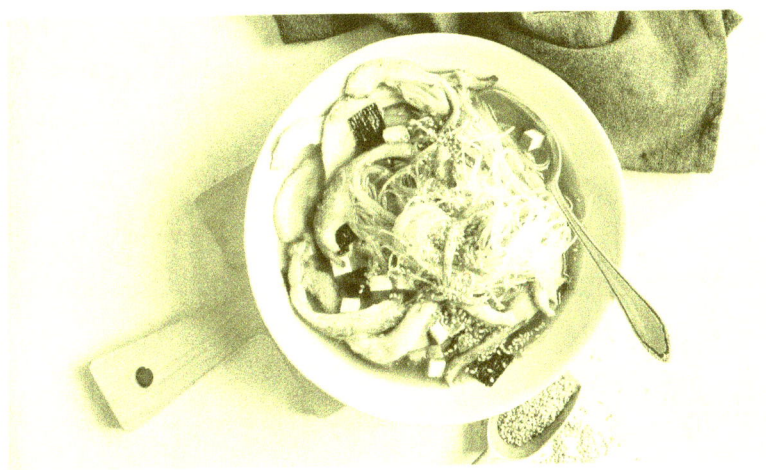

Ingredients:

- 15 g ginger
- 1.5 l Vegetable broth
- 4 tbsp Soy sauce
- 50 g dried (e.g. porcini mushrooms, morels, chanterelles mushrooms

- 100 g Glass noodles
- 150 g Smoked tofu
- 300 g Oyster mushrooms
- 1 sheet Nori
- 2 tbsp sesame
- 3 tbsp sesame oil
- salt

Peel the ginger and cut into thin slices. Cook with the dried mushrooms, vegetable stock and soy sauce in a closed saucepan for about 15 minutes over medium heat. At the end of the cooking time, pour the broth through a fine sieve, squeezing out the residue in the sieve well.

Put glass noodles in a large bowl and pour boiling water over them. Let it steep for a few minutes, drain through a fine sieve and drain well, possibly cut a little smaller with kitchen scissors.

Cut the smoked tofu into small cubes. Clean the oyster mushrooms and cut into fine strips. Cut the seaweed into small squares with scissors.

Briefly toast the sesame seeds in a non-stick frying pan until they smell fragrant. Put on a plate and let cool down briefly. Heat the sesame oil in the pan and briefly fry the oyster mushrooms and season with salt.

Briefly bring the broth to the boil again, add the tofu cubes and remove the soup from the stove. Spread the pasta, mushrooms and seaweed on 4 deep plates or bowls and fill up with the hot soup. Serve sprinkled with sesame seeds.

Quark breakfast with mango

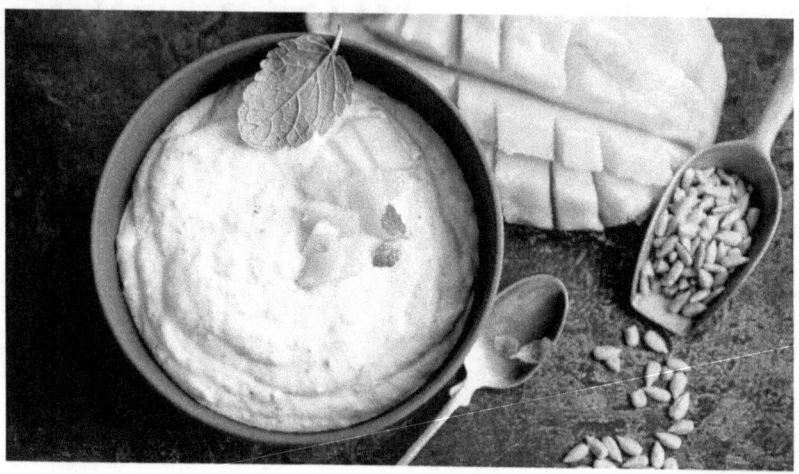

Ingredients:

- 0.5 mango
- 250 glow fat quark
- 3 tbsp Oat drink
- 1 tbsp linseed
- 1 tsp Flea seeds
- 1 tbsp Sunflower seeds
- 1 tbsp linseed oil

Peel the mango and remove the pulp from the stone. Put together with all other ingredients in a mixing bowl and puree until smooth with the mixer.

Nutritional values per serving:

431 kcal, 18 g fat, 25 g carbohydrates, 40 g protein, 8 g fiber, 2.1 BE

Quinoa bowl with tofu in sesame crust and broccoli

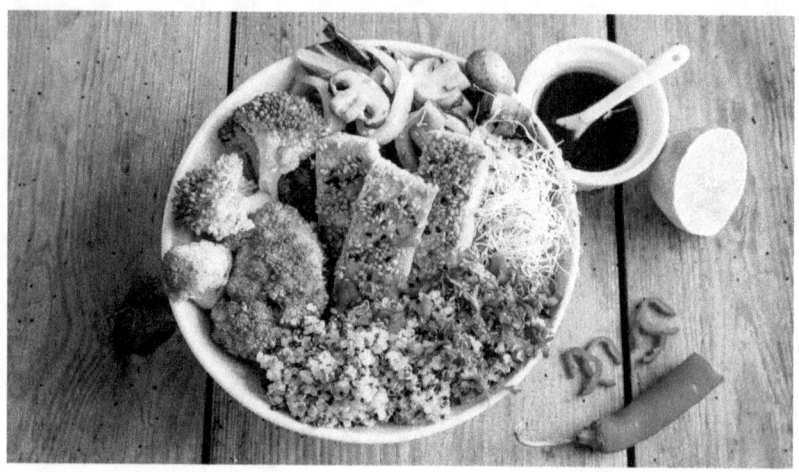

Ingredients:

- 200 g Quinoa
- 200 g Natural tofu
- 2 tbsp light sesame
- 2 tbsp black sesame
- 2 tbsp Coconut oil
- 200 g broccoli
- 1 smaller fennel
- 6th(e.g. shiitake or mushrooms) mushrooms
- 4 sheetsSwiss chard
- 1 handfularugula
- 40 gsliced almonds
- 2 tbsp Yeast flakes
- 1 handful Sprouts

- 1 red chilli pepper
- 2 stems parsley

Boil quinoa in double the amount of water and cook for 15 minutes over low heat with the lid closed. Then let it soak for at least 5 minutes.

While the quinoa is cooking, divide the cleaned broccoli into florets and steam in water. Cut the tofu into 1 cm thick slices. Mix the sesame seeds in a plate and turn the tofu slices in it. Heat the oil in a pan and fry the tofu on both sides over a medium heat for 5 minutes until crispy.

In the meantime, clean the fennel, mushrooms and Swiss chard and cut into bite-sized pieces. Take the tofu out of the pan and keep warm, heat the remaining oil, fry the vegetables and mushrooms in it for 5 minutes.

Wash the sprouts, rocket, chilli and parsley, chop the chilli and parsley.

Drain the broccoli, turn off the stove. Arrange the quinoa, tofu, vegetables, herbs, almonds and sprouts in the bowls, sprinkle with yeast flakes.

Nutritional values per serving:

990 kcal, 49 g fat, 86 g carbohydrates, 51 g protein, 21 g fiber, 7 BE, 8 mg zinc

Ingredients for the dressing:

- 1 tbsp Rape seed oil
- 2 tsp Soy sauce
- alternatively: Tamani
- 1 lime
- 1 tsp Liquid honey
- pepper

Squeeze the lime. Add the juice to the pan along with all the other ingredients for the dressing and toss briefly.

Pour the dressing over the bowls.

Nutritional values per serving:
990 kcal, 49 g fat, 86 g carbohydrates, 51 g protein, 21 g fiber, 8 mg zinc, 7 BE

Rice congee (Asian congee)

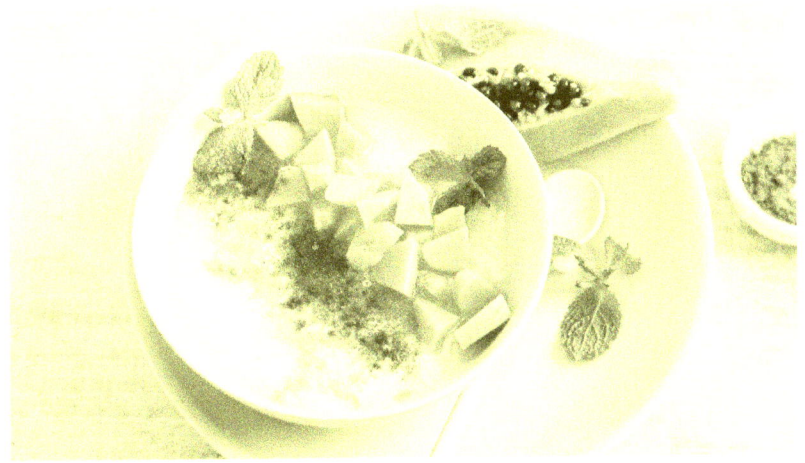

Ingredients:

- 50 g Basmati rice
- 0.5 l water
- 0.5 papaya
- 1 tsp cinnamon
- turmeric

Wash the rice thoroughly, bring to the boil with water and cook in an open pot for 20 minutes. Then simmer for at least 1 hour over the lowest heat with the lid on. Put in a bowl.

Remove the pulp from the papaya and dice. Pour over the rice porridge together with the spices.

Tip:

Congee can be eaten for breakfast with fresh or dried fruit (such as dates), but also as a hearty meal with some vegetables such as fennel and carrots.

Nutritional values per serving:

234 kcal, 1 g fat, 50 g carbohydrates, 5 g protein, 5 g fiber, 4 BE

Pollack on creamed spinach

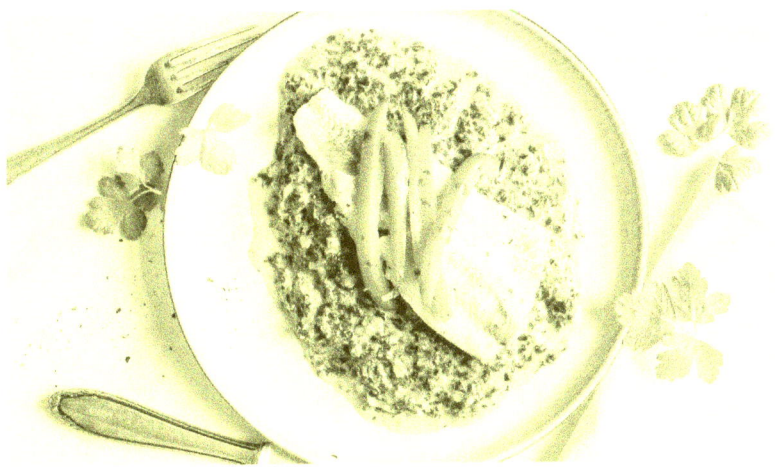

Ingredients:

- 100 g Pollack fillet
- 50 gred pepper
- 1 small Shallot
- 1 tbsp Rapeseed oil
- 100 g Frozen spinach
- 1 tbsp low-fat cream cheese
- 2 tbsp (15% fat) cooking cream
- nutmeg
- salt
- pepper

Wash the pollack and pat dry. Wash and core the peppers and cut into fine strips.

Peel the shallot, cut into fine cubes and sauté with rapeseed oil in a saucepan. Add spinach and let thaw on low heat. Add the cream cheese and cream and season with nutmeg, salt and pepper.

Put the saithe on the spinach and lightly salt. Place the pepper strips on the saithe. With the lid closed, let everything simmer for about 5 minutes on a medium setting.

To do this, consume a potato if you like.

Nutritional values (per serving):
approx. 285 kcal, 24 g protein, 8 g carbohydrates, 18 g fat, 3 g fiber

Comprehensive & Useful Tips

A herpes attack is painful and unsightly, but it is also accompanied by a very significant risk of contamination of those around you. As soon as the warning signs of a herpes attack (tingling, itching, burning sensations, numbness, pain ??), the risk of transmission of the virus is high, even before the formation of clumps of vesicles, which are filled with a liquid that contains the virus.

Avoid contact at the first signs

During the warning signs and during the crisis, it is therefore advisable to avoid all direct contact such as kissing in case of cold sore and sexual relations in case of genital herpes. On the treatment side, we do not know how to cure herpes. On the other hand, there is an antiviral (aciclovir and valaciclovir) capable of reducing the frequency of herpes attacks and their intensity.

1. Consult

When in doubt, consult (attending physician, dermatologist, gynecologist or urologist) and preferably during a herpes attack in order to facilitate the diagnosis, to cure the current crisis more quickly and to limit contagion.

2. Identify your own triggering factors

This in order to limit the frequency of your attacks, to take your preventive treatment as soon as possible and again to limit contagion: stress, sun exposure, alcohol consumption, fatigue, fever, menstruation. Menstrual periods, local trauma, etc.

3. Look for the warning signs of a herpes attack

4. If you come into contact with a lesion, wash yourself

After contact with the lesions, wash your hands systematically to avoid contamination of another part of the body or those around you. Obviously, avoid touching or scratching the lesions and do not touch your eyes (risk of ocular herpes).

5. Clean affected areas

Keep **affected** areas clean by washing them with soap and water and then drying them (hair dryer on low heat if necessary).

6. Avoid bandages

Avoid bandaging lesions as they heal better in the open. On the other hand, during short moments of essential contact (such as taking care of a small child), it is possible to use a waterproof bandage to reinforce the precautionary measures.

7. Do not share your towel or toothbrush

8. Herpes labialis

- Avoid kissing, talking too closely and spitting especially in the presence of a newborn baby, a pregnant woman, people with atopic eczema or any other subject with weakened immune defenses.

- Likewise, do not exchange your cutlery and everyone drinks from their glass.
- Avoid oral-genital sex because a cold sore can lead to genital herpes and vice versa.

9. Genital herpes

- Use a condom during sex. Abstinence is sometimes recommended during relapses (to avoid contamination, spread and also because intercourse can become painful). It is best to discuss this with your doctor.
- Pregnant women should report any outbreak of genital herpes to their doctor.
- Avoid wearing tight clothing (jeans, tights ??) and synthetic underwear to limit humidity.

Conclusion

In conclusion, herpes genitals has become one of the most common sexually transmitted diseases and has reached epidemic proportions. It presents a grave risk to immune compromised patients and to newborns. The advent of effective therapy with acyclovir has dramatically modified the morbidity and mortality of disseminated herpes virus infection and has helped in the therapy of primary and recurrent herpes genitals. Current work has indicated that the disease can be transmitted by asymptomatic patients who are shedding the virus in the absence of visible lesions, which presents a diagnostic and therapeutic problem, especially significant for the pregnant patient, because infection of the neonate leads to serious consequences. Close follow-up of the pregnant woman with genital herpes therefore is imperative to minimize the risk to the newborn. At this time, no vaccines have been demonstrated to be safe and effective; therefore, prevention is of the utmost importance.

www.ingramcontent.com/pod-product-compliance
Lightning Source LLC
Chambersburg PA
CBHW050250220526
45465CB00002B/620